I0116978

WHO ARE YOU CALLING OBESE?

One Woman's Triumph over Obesity and Food Addiction

Gwen Allman

Published by

King Arthur Publishing
Yorktown, VA
TeamAllman.com

This book is a motivational tool only and not intended to be a substitute for sound medical advice. Please consult your physician before starting any diet or exercise program.

Copyright © 2016 by Gwendolyn Allman
Published by
King Arthur Publishing
Yorktown, VA
TeamAllman.com

All rights reserved. No part of this book may be reproduced or transmitted in any form or by any means, electronic or mechanical, without prior written consent of the publisher, except for the inclusion of brief quotes in a review. Thank you for your support of the author's rights.

ISBN: 0998201200
ISBN: 9780998201207
Library of Congress Control Number: 2016919185

Front and Back Cover Design by Karen Walker Designs
Edited by Tenita Johnson, So It Is Written, LLC
Author's photo by Timorah Beales Photography

Printed in the United States of America

WHAT PEOPLE ARE SAYING . . .

"Wow!! Gwen delivers a knockout punch right out of the gate. Great job in capturing a lot of women's "truth"! Thank you for lighting a spark in many of us to do better. Feed me more…"

~ Karen Y. Smith, Systems Analyst

"Gwen has used her life story to motivate others. I saw her transformation firsthand. She doesn't just talk about it; she lives her life about it! Her love of life and sense of humor (even in the hardest times) have pushed her to achieve success. Allow her story to inspire and help transform you!"

~Charlotte Rucker, Owner of Celebration Creations Cakes and Catering

"I have had the pleasure of knowing Gwen for over 20 years. She is one of those rare, quiet leaders-- who when faced with a challenge, does so with strength and vision. I am so inspired by her willingness to lift people up through this book. It has been something special for me to watch her evolve and blossom into the absolutely amazing woman she is today!!!"

~Sharon D. Howard, Office of Public and Community Relations at Miami Valley Hospital

"Gwen is an unforgettable friend, a sister entrepreneur, and a lover of the Light. Her kindness, love, and graceful living have been and continue to be her "signature". And now, with this new endeavor, the written word in her own words, she has the opportunity to bring the beauty that is inside her outside for the entire world to see, learn, and appreciate. So please... read, learn, and grow to know this gifted one."

~Missy Duer, 6th generation entrepreneur, Historic Staley Mill Farm & Indian Creek Distillery
New Carlisle, Ohio

"I think sharing is the best way to heal. Conquering obstacles leads to triumphs that are explored and communicated; and the resulting emotional response rejuvenates the soul. Gwen Allman is the navigator when it comes to resilience and tenacity. She can give you the tools to successfully commute your own journey."

~Marsha Bonhart, Director of Development for Dayton Contemporary Dance Company and former News Anchor/Reporter at NBC news affiliate, WDTN-TV

ACKNOWLEDGMENTS

To my Heavenly Father, who purposefully allowed my journey to include people who brought overwhelming disappointment, grief and pain. Thank you for these valuable lessons. I learned them well. I am strong today because of the heartbreak I endured.

Heartfelt thanks to my editor, Tenita Johnson of So It Is Written LLC, for your expertise, time, and patience with me. As a virgin writer, I was so intimidated by the whole process. Your keen eye, sweet spirit, professionalism, and sense of humor were both comforting and refreshing to me.

To Valerie J. Lewis-Coleman, Pen of the Writer, LLC, you are an amazing human being. Your tireless efforts to encourage aspiring writers have been a well of inspiration to me along this journey. Thank you.

I'd like to send a huge shout out to Dr. Eric McHenry, my family physician of so many years. I cannot thank you enough for your honesty and professionalism. I am indebted to you for my success in conquering obesity, overcoming depression, and so many other issues that threatened my health and well-being.

To Dr. Barry Taylor, my Mother's physician, thank you for all you did to help her. She adored you.

Thank you to Professor Jamey Dunham, my English teacher at Sinclair Community College. You were one of the first teachers who encouraged me to publish my writings. Little did you know how much I needed those encouraging words. Your timing could not have been more perfect. I totally love you. Your classes were some of my best times at SCC.

To Professor Kathleen Querner, thank you for believing in me and giving me an internship I will never forget. I am so in awe of you.

How do I begin to say "Thank you" to my children? You loved and supported me when I didn't know how to love myself. I pray that my decision to make my health a priority will result in many more years of me being able to be an active part of your futures. Thank you for following in my footsteps and making physical fitness and a healthy diet such an integral part of your lives.

Thank you to my grandchildren, who inspire me to set a healthy example of wholesome living. May you continue the legacy of Team Allman to the next generation and beyond.

To my best friend, Claudia, you've been with me every step of the way. You've been my lifeline and like a sister to me for too many years to count. You've held me down when I thought I was coming apart. Thank you for your unconditional love for me. I love you dearly.

To my Power Team, and all those who believed in me, prayed for me, and encouraged me to write my story, "Thank you". You know who you are.

DEDICATION

To My Children and Grandchildren
Eric, Jasmeen, Anthony, Christian, Noelle,
Eric II and Aubrey
"You are the reason I live"

Rest in Peace
Mother and Daddy
"Forever in my heart"

Rest in Peace
Zion
"My fur baby"

TABLE OF CONTENTS

INTRODUCTION

I can almost bet money that if you are reading this, you are either an obese person or you know someone who is. If the former is true, it's safe to say that you have either already received a formal diagnosis from your physician, or you at least suspect that your recent health problems might be linked to your excessive weight.

Whether you have admitted it or not, you have finally come to the conclusion that you can no longer ignore your weight issue. You are overwhelmed, frustrated with yourself, and scared. But, there is good news: you are not alone. Between 2009 and 2010, more than 35% of American men and women, 20 years and older, were obese. Seventeen percent of children, ages 2-19, were also obese. (Ogden, Carroll and Kit) Obesity is the second leading cause of preventable death in the United States. It is still on the rise.

In 2009, I was diagnosed as obese. My doctor told me that if I didn't lose weight, I would eventually have a heart attack or stroke and die. If by some chance I lived, doctors said that my quality of life would suffer greatly unless I made changes to my diet and lifestyle. When I asked my doctor to give it to me straight, I had no idea that he would tell me such disturbing news. Even still, it took me an entire year after the diagnosis before I did anything about my weight or lifestyle.

At the time of my diagnosis, I was a single mother, working in corporate America. Overwhelmed with the stress of juggling both a career and home, I turned to food for comfort. I sat at a desk all day and snacked constantly. Most days, I was overwhelmed with telephone calls from disgruntled customers. Work commitments obligated me to dine out often with potential clients in the evenings. Mandatory overtime took up most of my weekends.

At home, I maintained the same insane workload, with kids involved in sports and extra-curricular activities. I rarely had any time to relax, let alone focus on my own needs and health. Although I ran around like crazy, I never purposely set aside time to follow an exercise program for its health benefits. I exercised twice a week as part of my company's wellness program, but my heart wasn't into it. I didn't expect results. I did it as a way to get out of the office for a few hours each week.

Being obese is one of the most difficult things to overcome. Admitting it is even more difficult. No one wants to admit that their excessive body weight might lead to an untimely death. We avoid the subject of death like the plague. We would rather not talk about it. We curse ourselves for even thinking about it. We would much rather cover it up or postpone the conversation until a later date. Family and friends, though concerned, do not want to appear rude or insensitive. Although each moment spent in an obese body is pure hell on earth, somehow, we fool ourselves into believing that we can handle being miserable and uncomfortable. We hope and pray that it will work itself out if we just ignore the facts.

We go to great lengths to deny that there is anything wrong with the unhealthy lifestyle we live from day to day. We surround ourselves with people that act and look just like us. We allow friends and family to lie to us and appease us. They tell us that they love us just the way we are. We choose to ignore the warning signals that cry out from our bodies. Instead, we convince ourselves that we possess self-love, just not enough to go to the doctor, or to educate ourselves about what is going on with our health. We live in the fast lane of a "Que sera sera" lifestyle until we are stuffed into a pine box, leaving behind a host of guilt-ridden family and friends who were too afraid to speak up and tell us the truth.

Obesity is not cute or trendy. It is not fashionable. But if you are obese, it does not have to be a death sentence. There is something you can do about it. But, you will have to put in some serious work to reverse it. Others can encourage, educate and inspire you, but the fight is ultimately yours and yours alone. It is going to take everything that is in you to overcome this food addiction. You will feel like giving up a lot of the time, but you must keep moving forward.

This fight is not for the weak, the wimpy, the faint or the wishy-washy. This fight is for the warrior, the crazy, the insane, the dare-to-be-different person--the person who is beyond ready for a change, the person who has everything to live for and wants to win just as bad as he or she wants to take the next breath. If you are that person, then welcome to the battleground. In the end, you win.

If you are not the person I just described, then please put this book down and walk away. By doing so, you admit that you are not ready for change. You have to be okay with that. Reading any further would simply be a waste of your time. My mission here is not to gain popularity by telling you that as long as you are happy in your obese state, it's okay. My mission is to get so far underneath your skin with the truth that you will be uncomfortable enough to change, even if you're angry at me in the end. After reading my story, I want to hear you say, "She told the truth. She kept it real, and it saved my life."

1

"The truth will set you free. But first,
it will piss you off."

-Gloria Steinem

When my doctor told me that I was obese, I wanted to slap him across the room. Immediately, I was offended. My first thought was, "Who are you calling obese?"

I suppressed my inner Tasmanian devil long enough to ask, "What do you mean I'm obese? Are you sure you have the right chart?"

He nodded and explained that the excess fat I was carrying attributed to the trouble I experienced with my knees.

"The recommended weight for your height is right around 140 pounds," he said. "Anything over that is going to cause considerable damage to your knees over time."

He also mentioned something about my BMI being over 30 and concerns with my family history.

"Since you have a family history of obesity, diabetes, heart disease and cancer, you have a much greater risk of developing these same conditions if your weight is left unchecked," he explained.

He could have been speaking gibberish for all I know. My inner Taz was pitching a hissy fit so loud that I couldn't hear a word he was saying.

Somewhere between my doctor's lengthy explanation and him handing me the American Heart Association diet plan, I must have zoned out. The next thing I knew, he was walking out the door and the nurse was asking me if I had any questions. I heard myself say, "No," but inside, I was dying to know what the hell had just happened. I was seeking answers for my constant knee pain, knee collapses, aching back and shortness of breath. Truthfully, I had actually come seeking sympathy with a dose of compassion on the side. I sure as hell was not satisfied with the answer or the treatment plan I received.

I hurriedly put on my clothes and stomped out to the check-out counter to pay my co-pay. I was livid! The mere thought that I had to pay this man after he had insulted me angered me even more. Hell, I already knew I was fat. But obese...those were fighting words!

My anger continued out into the parking lot, where I briefly glanced at the American Heart Association diet plan before depositing it into the nearest trash can. All I could think about was how ticked off I was and how bad I needed something sweet. Luckily, there was a gas station nearby. I was able to appease my appetite and my attitude with a low-calorie blueberry muffin, a double latte and a chocolate candy bar for later.

Don't get me wrong; I love my doctor. He's been there for me more than thirty years. I value his opinion and trust his judgment. But this time, I thought he was exaggerating just a tad. Had I really heard him say, "Either lose the weight or risk dying?" He must have had a rough night with the Mrs. or got up on the wrong side of the bed that morning. There was no way I was obese.

As I drove home, I thought about what lie I would tell my children. I certainly wouldn't let them know I'd been diagnosed as obese. They'd had enough bad news to last a lifetime.

Several years prior, I'd lost my mother to complications from morbid obesity. Her doctor called it Pickwickian syndrome, a hypoventilation disorder that causes an extremely obese person to stop breathing for short periods of time while sleeping. The resulting poor quality of sleep often leads to excessive drowsiness during the day. This, in turn, puts a considerable amount of strain on the heart. Massive heart attacks and strokes are inevitable, and they lead to death in most cases. Congestive heart failure and respiratory issues are also common.

Her struggle, and subsequent death, took a toll on all of us. My children witnessed firsthand the anger and frustration I felt toward her for not doing anything about her weight. How hypocritical would it seem to them if I were heading down that same path? At the time, it was so easy for me to judge her. Now, I found it extremely hard to admit I was becoming her.

So I took my little secret, wrapped it up in a box, neatly tucked it away in the back of my mind, and decided to do absolutely nothing with it. As a matter of fact, I walked into the house that day and boldly stated that I was just fine.

"It's arthritis, guys. Nothing major."

2

As much as I hate to admit it, I have watched, and even at times, enjoyed, The Steve Wilkos Show. It's one of those raunchy, drama-filled, late-night talk shows where couples take lie detector tests to find out if one of them is cheating. After Steve reads the results, the cheating partner insists that the results are wrong, and asks for another test. Keep in mind that the test is administered multiple times before the show airs. The lengths to which the cheater goes in order to prove his innocence makes for pretty entertaining, late-night TV.

The over-the-top drama and pseudo-physical violence usually escalates to the point that Steve will call the examiner to the stage. The examiner rattles off his credentials, and explains to the live audience that the test is 99.9% accurate; however, the guilty party will swear on his or her mama's grave that the lie detector test is faulty. I can't tell you how many times I have yelled at the TV and harrumphed about the cheater being in total denial. But this is exactly how I behaved about my obesity diagnosis. Vehemently, I denied it, hoping that it would go away. Maybe it would if I kept saying it wasn't true.

I desperately wanted to make another appointment with my doctor to be weighed again. This time, I planned to remove my shoes, earrings, bracelets--anything that may cause a misreading on the scale. I'd be sure to remind the nurse that clothes account for some of the pounds you see on the scale. Heck, I'd insist on being weighed naked, if need be. I'd even seek a second opinion, if push came to shove. I just needed someone to tell me that I was not obese and apologize for the error. I read somewhere that medical mistakes happen more often than we realize. I wanted them to lie to me, if necessary. I just didn't want them to call me the "O" word.

I come from a long line of women with big breasts, thick waistlines and wide hips. My mother, grandmother and aunts were all large women. So it was no surprise that I was big. Other than my mother, I had never heard of anyone else in my circle being labeled as obese. Practically, everyone I knew was overweight to some degree, and they never mentioned the word obese. If they were, they certainly weren't talking about it.

That word, and all that it implies, was something I just could not handle. It hurt. It cut deep. The fat lady at the circus was obese. People paid her to be a freak of nature. I knew I was not *that* big. I had convinced myself over the years that I was just a little thick. I told myself that I was a tad bit overweight, big-boned, curvy and bloated...anything, but obese. After all, there is nothing wrong with having a little meat on the bones or a little junk in the trunk.

Having a big butt is even considered fashionable by Hollywood's standards. Women pay money for the size butt that I had. Have you seen JLo, Kim Kardashian or Nicki Minaj? Their big behinds are what made them filthy rich!

I stayed angry for weeks after my visit to the doctor. For weeks, I treated myself to as many comfort foods as I could consume. I packed on another five to 10 pounds, at least. I was an emotional eater. I ate when I was mad, sad, glad or just bad. Everything I did revolved around food.

Cultures are defined by their cuisine and feasting. Breaking bread is a good thing. It is totally acceptable to celebrate with food. The Food Network was birthed out of our obsession with food, eating and cooking. Although my mind kept coming up with legitimate reasons for my excessive food consumption, I couldn't get over the fact that my doctor had actually come out and said, "You are obese." You just don't go around calling people obese.

Finally, I had to ask myself why I couldn't get over this. What was it about the word *obesity* that triggered all of this rage in me? Why wasn't the "sticks-and-stones-may-break my-bones, but-words-will-never-hurt-me" chant working for me? To agree with my doctor's diagnosis, I would have to admit my dysfunction. Who wants to look in the mirror and tell themselves the unadulterated truth?

"You are beyond fat, sister. You are obese. You *are* the fat lady!" I mockingly said aloud, in my Maury Povich voice.

I just could not admit that. How dare my doctor blatantly expose my dysfunction! Too often, I'd heard myself say, "She ought to be ashamed of herself for wearing that outfit. She knew when she put that on, it was too tight. Does she not have mirrors in her house?" If it was an obese man, I'd say to myself, "If he doesn't take off that stupid-looking tie! He's so big!

He doesn't even have a neck. Where's his neck? I don't see a neck. Do you see a neck?"

I have ridiculed, poked fun at, and made obese people the butt of many of my funniest jokes. I was just having fun, though. I didn't mean any harm by it. The thought that some-one may have said some of these same things about me was heartbreaking. I did not look that big, though. Why would my mirror lie to me?

I dressed up my dysfunction for so many years. I wore "good" clothes. Everybody knows when you wear "good" clothes; you can fit into a size 18 when you are really a size 22.

My mother taught me to shop in the upscale stores for quality fabrics like silk, wool, cashmere and knit. I was the self-appointed Spanx® Queen. I kept my fat wrapped, strapped, locked and blocked. It didn't wiggle or jiggle. Sometimes, I was wrapped so tightly under my clothes, I struggled to breathe. But that is the price I paid to look good.

I kept my hair fried, dyed and laid to the side. My feet and nails were always done. My makeup was impeccable. I spent so much time in the mirror that my college roommate called me "Marilyn Monroe." I followed a strict regimen of cleansing, toning, exfoliation, masks and moisturizers. I popped Hair, Skin and Nails® gummies like they were candy.

Guys told me I had a pretty face. Some even called me gor-geous a few times. Admittedly, I didn't get many compliments on my body, but most of my friends and family were the same size or bigger than I was. So it really didn't matter that much. I always felt confident about my appearance--except for that one time in high school when I overheard a group of pimply-faced boys say I looked like a refrigerator from behind. What the heck did they know anyway? After all, it was high school.

I must admit, I was devastated at the time, though. I carried the sting of those words into adulthood; however, I learned ways to cope whenever that little incident came to mind. Although my doctor had come in like a wrecking ball and totally shattered my monument of denial, I assured myself that with a little effort, it should not be hard to get over the pain of his words either.

3

I read somewhere that if you need motivation to lose weight, avoiding death is probably a good reason. Although I lived with constant knee and back pain, I was not motivated to lose weight. After having kids, I gained so much weight that losing it seemed like an insurmountable task.

In my mind, a constant battle raged over exercising, dieting, dying and living. Most times, it felt like I was on a speeding freight train, heading toward a concrete wall. No matter how much I wanted to jump off--fully aware of the destruction and possible death that lie ahead--I just couldn't get off the train, or my butt, for that matter.

I had been in a funk since my mother passed away. Six months prior to that, I lost my dad to stomach cancer. I was going through life on autopilot. I was existing, but not really living. I wore my mask well, keeping myself as busy as possible with work, my business and taking care of home. On the inside though, the funeral dirge was quietly playing.

I constantly daydreamed, replaying my mother's final days. Was there something I could have done differently? Was there something I could have said to make her want to live? Why did I not stay with her the night she was admitted into the ER and coded? Why did I not just ignore the DNR she had requested, and let the paramedics resuscitate her? Why? Why? Why?

Burned into my psyche were images of her being hoisted up on a crane-like contraption, just to be put into a wheelchair to go to the bathroom. It reminded me of a news report I saw. A stray cow, who was lost in the woods, had to be air-lifted by helicopter back to its pasture. I will never forget the image of that cow being hoisted higher and higher into the air.

It seemed so inhumane for my mother to be treated like an animal, but she couldn't get up on her own. Sometimes, it took two or three of us just to get her in an upright position. Putting her into a wheelchair was nearly impossible.

I remembered how exhausting it was to roll her over to change her diaper or give her a bath. The endless days of dressing that gaping wound on her stomach, caused by a feeding tube disaster, caused constant flashbacks in my mind.

For seven months, I slept in the ICU and emergency rooms of Miami Valley Hospital, area nursing homes, and home at my mother's bedside. All of my prayers, faith confessions and reverse psychology tricks were not enough to motivate her to live. She was overwhelmed by her diagnosis. Unfortunately, being morbidly obese was not the only issue she had. Diabetes, sleep apnea, congestive heart failure, kidney failure, pneumonia, incontinence and feelings of hopelessness all accompanied the excessive weight gain. She got tired of fighting what seemed like a losing battle. She welcomed death and the release from agony that only it could bring.

There were days, in that nursing home, that I was so angry at my mother that I walked out of the room. I pleaded with her to just try to move some, to get up and join the others in the activity group. I knew it was too much to expect from someone so grossly overweight, but I just needed her to do something other than lie there and give up.

I decorated her room with bright colors, pictures and cards. I kept the Scripture, set to music, playing quietly in her room in hopes of breaking through the never-ending bouts of depression she experienced most days. I constantly reminded her that we needed her, especially since Daddy was gone. I told her how much her grandchildren needed her. I preached to her that being obese was not a legitimate reason to die. It was like preaching to a brick wall.

When my mother's doctor told me there was nothing else he could do for her, I was totally blindsided.

"So, you're telling me my mother is going to die?" I asked, utterly confused.

"Your mother wants to die; therefore, she will die," her doctor replied softly.

"How can that be? She is morbidly obese. How is that a terminal illness?"

"I have been advising your mother about her health for many years now, and she has not done a single thing I have asked her to do in regards to her diabetes, weight or managing her stress. She is extremely depressed and does not have the will to live. Your mother is who she is. It is her life and her decision to make. I cannot override her will and force her to want to live or to take care of herself. And neither can you," he earnestly explained.

"But isn't there something you can give her, or at least talk to her again? We just lost our dad. We can't lose our mother, too. She loves you, Dr. Taylor. Couldn't you just talk to her one more time?" I pleaded in utter desperation.

After a long pause, he agreed to stop by the next day and talk to my mother. Though relieved, I couldn't shake the apprehension I felt as I left his office. I could accept death by natural cause. I could accept death by cancer, heart attack or stroke. But I could not, I would not, accept death by gluttony.

I raced home to my mother's bedside to tell her the good news.

"Guess who's coming to see you tomorrow, Mother?" I asked, plopping down beside her on the bed.

When she didn't answer, I enthusiastically announced, "Dr. Taylor!"

That got a weak smile out of her, but nothing more.

My mother died in the pre-dawn hours of the next day. I sometimes think she purposely slipped away when no one was watching. I honestly believe she wanted to avoid having to listen to another speech about why she should fight to live. Even in death, she was going to have things her way.

Dr. Taylor was right. Often, I am reminded of the conversation I had with him. He probably knew her better than any of us. I am sure she opened up to him about her desperation and fears. I just wish she had shared them with me.

As I bathed my mother's lifeless body for the last time, I turned to Ellen, her hospice nurse, and said, "She looks so peaceful. I guess she's happy now."

"I'm sure she is," Ellen replied softly.

Time has not erased the image of that black leather body bag being wheeled through the living room of my mother's home, nor the hearse driving away as we stood sobbing on the sidewalk. Nothing prepares us to lose our parents. Nothing.

I swore at my mother's funeral that I would never cause my children and grandchildren the depth of pain she caused me. I didn't think I would ever be able to forgive her for leaving us the way she did. I literally couldn't function after she died. For days after her funeral, I couldn't get out of bed. I couldn't eat. I couldn't think straight. There were times that I could not breathe. It took every ounce of strength I had to brush my teeth and comb my hair. Her death paralyzed me. I became so numb. I honestly didn't know if I was coming or going. It felt like an elephant was sitting on my chest with no plans of getting up any time soon.

4

"Imitation is the sincerest [form] of flattery."

-Charles Caleb Colton

After my mother died, very few things brought me pleasure. It was like I was in a fog with no way out. It is the nature of fog to completely surround you, to cause total blindness and consume you with overwhelming fear. Although your eyes are wide open, it is impossible to see in the fog. Your mind races with panic. Your heart rate increases, eyes dilate, and your palms become sweaty. As you cautiously navigate forward, you can never know for sure if something is in front of you, in back of you or beside you. You instinctively slow down and proceed with extreme caution. Sometimes, it feels safer to not move at all because you are so fearful of crashing into what lies ahead.

My days of living in the fog were plagued by highs and lows. However, the one thing that remained constant was my obsession with keeping my mother's spirit, memory and traditions alive. She was best known for her extravagant cooking style. She was a master chef and baker. She was the queen of all things culinary. I became obsessed with entertaining family and friends, reaching back into my childhood and pulling out all the old recipes I could remember. It was like I was taken over by her spirit every time I prepared one of her extraordinary meals.

Sunday dinners were always happy times when I was growing up. My parents prepared these enormous buffets, which were fit for royalty. Daddy barbecued in the backyard, and my mother cooked in the kitchen. We didn't lack for much in the way of food because my dad was a gardener extraordinaire, a hunter, and a self-proclaimed grill master. All three of our deep freezers looked like the meat aisle of the grocery store. Every year, he had a whole cow butchered and packaged so that we would have plenty of meat to freeze and plenty to share with others. He grew all of the vegetables and most of the fruit we enjoyed year-round.

My mother's food presentation was nothing short of a madrigal feast. It didn't have to be a special occasion for her to prepare one of her spectacular buffets. The pantry was always crammed with delights and delicacies that she painstakingly canned herself. She also grew magnificent fresh flowers to garnish her food platters and she created lush edible centerpieces for her tablescapes. Imitating her and recreating those Sunday dinners seemed to be the only thing that brought me joy and some resemblance of normalcy.

Quickly, my need for feasts, family and friends took over my life. I filled my calendar with social events where food was the main focus. Brunches, lunches, dinners and cookouts--if food was being served, I was there. If there was no event to attend, I would host my own. I was constantly in the kitchen, preparing cakes, cookies, cheesecakes, Friendship bread, date nut bread, banana pudding and tea cakes. This was just the dessert portion of the meals I prepared.

On the main menu were BBQ ribs, southern fried chicken, turkey and dressing, pork chops, chitterlings, macaroni and cheese, collard greens, mashed potatoes and gravy, string beans, fried corn, fried green tomatoes and okra, homemade yeast rolls and jalapeño cornbread. I always prepared enough for an army. You better believe an army of friends and family is what I got when word got out that I was in the kitchen.

I even got the kids involved. I created a small business for them called *Angel Treats*. We specialized in snack-attack gift bags. We dipped pretzel rods in white or milk chocolate and rolled them in Reese's peanut butter chips or toffee bits. We baked giant chocolate chip cookies with nuts to go with the pretzel rods. To that, we added a package of microwave kettle corn, wrapped everything up nicely in a gift bag, and sold these packaged treats to friends and family. To the outside world, I handled everything just fine. Martha Stewart would have been proud to have me on her team.

Secretly, I was feeding my grief, tasting as much during the cooking process as I was eating during the actual meal. My plate always resembled a mini mountain, with layers upon layers of delicious food, artistically arranged and jam-packed onto a 10-inch, gold-rimmed china plate.

It's funny how the pre-dinner prayer always mentioned something about nourishing our bodies when I was doing everything but that. No one dared say a word about the weight I gained though. Everyone knows, as long as Mom is happy, so is everyone else.

5

I can't quite put my finger on the exact moment I realized something was grossly wrong with this picture. Somewhere between the time people started telling me I was beginning to look more and more like my mom and when I started wearing muumuus, I had an epiphany.

For those of you who are not familiar with muumuus, they are floor-length casual dresses that fat women wear to hide their bodies. They are usually floral-patterned or some other hideous design, loose-fitting, flowing, and made from polyester. I swore I would never be caught dead in a muumuu. Yet, here I stood "muumuu-ed down," gazing at my reflection in the mirror.

You never wear high heels with a muumuu. I'm not quite sure why. That is just the rule. Ballerina flats, flip flops, or some other kind of fancy house shoe was the acceptable choice. The muumuu was all about comfort, ease of movement and disguise. You could hide a person under a muumuu, and no one would even know it.

Accessories were also important when wearing the muumuu. Everything had to be large. Not just large, but huge. The bigger the earrings, the better. Necklaces had to be enormous or multilayered. Huge hair or some kind of matching head wrap always worked well, too. The accessories served one purpose: to draw attention away from the fact that you were wearing a giant trash bag.

So here I was, dressed in my muumuu of choice, when suddenly the thought came, "You look like a refrigerator."

It slithered in so quickly and quietly, I was blindsided by it. I found myself desperately gasping for air and clutching at my chest as I realized I actually did resemble a floral-printed Maytag!

Slowly I turned to the side, back and front. I was as wide as I was tall. The indent where my waistline used to be was long gone. Gravity was calling my stomach to the floor, and my stomach was answering the call.

What was this expansive protrusion of fat sitting underneath my breasts? Was it a second stomach? Why did I look like I was in my final trimester of pregnancy? For crying out loud, those idiots from high school were onto something!

My face was beautiful, though. Lord knows, I heard that enough times in my life. MAC® and Mary Kay® cosmetics had been good to me over the years. But whose body was this? And where in the hell was mine? HELP!

᠀

I can remember when I went away to college. I discovered my real body. For seventeen years, I had no idea I actually had a long, narrow boyish frame. Walking the hills on campus at Ohio University helped me drop a considerable amount of weight my freshman year. "She's Got Legs", by ZZ Top, was the theme song of my life in those days.

I also changed my diet as soon as I started college. The cafeteria wasn't serving up the kind of food I was used to eating. I actually enjoyed the vast selection of fresh fruit, vegetables and lean meats. Although it wasn't as well seasoned as my mom's cooking, the bland diet was filling, and I adapted quickly. I also discovered yogurt, skim milk, smoothies and other healthy goodies that I didn't have at home. It was the first time I experimented with salad as an entrée. I liked the way I felt after eating a meal. I didn't have any more food comas, just lots and lots of energy.

I even sought out new and creative ways to exercise by enrolling in several PE classes. I chose activities like tennis, swimming and yoga to balance out my challenging course load. With the beautiful Hocking Hills State Park just a short car drive away, it wasn't long before I was hiking the trails, canoeing and horseback riding. I discovered a whole new world. I discovered the endorphin high!

Never before had I connected food with energy or movement with mental clarity. I noticed that I felt light and energetic after a meal. My energy levels were through the roof after exercise. I fell in love with this new feeling, my new life, and my new body. By the end of my first year of college, I was wearing a size seven instead of a 14. I was the happiest I had been in a long time.

Unfortunately, that happiness was short-lived. When I moved back home for the summer, my mother wasn't happy with all the weight I lost. She certainly wasn't happy when I turned down the food she cooked. We battled like feral cats over my food choices and my new-found independence. She even marched me down to her doctor's office and told him I was anorexic. On the contrary, I felt better than I had in a long time, and I told him so. Poor man, he was caught in the middle of a battle he didn't want to be in. But he had to be truthful and tell her he couldn't find anything wrong with me, which only made matters worse. Needless to say, it was a long, long summer.

Standing in front of my mirror that day, caught up in the reverie of days gone by, yet paralyzed by the revelation that I did indeed look like a refrigerator, something broke inside of me. I started crying. I cried because I had become my mother. I cried because I knew she was never coming back, and I missed her terribly. I cried because I had chosen to ignore the fear I saw in my children's eyes as I picked up more weight. I cried because I felt so fat, so alone, so sad and so empty.

Hopelessness gripped me as I sank to the floor. Anger's arms embraced me as I curled up into a fetal position. Pain whispered to me that it was okay to die. Darkness engulfed my soul as I willed myself to just let go and be no more. Tears flowed down my face and formed puddles on the floor beside my head. I wept uncontrollably because the person staring back at me in the mirror was my mother.

In that moment, I knew her pain.

6

What most people fail to understand about obesity is that you do not get as big as I got without going through some serious pain. The false assumption is that obese people are just lazy, gluttonous, and too stupid to practice moderation. That theory is all wrong. I know from personal experience that people get this way because of deep pain and mishandling of that pain.

Obese people are masters at suppressing hurt and pain. The secrets we keep buried inside of us are often too hideous to share with anyone. So they lie dormant until something or someone triggers that memory. The wound reopens and festers, poisoning us from within. In our quest to appear unscathed to the perpetrators of the pain, we turn to food to satiate our physical and emotional needs. Our lives become a vicious cycle of pain, suppression and satiation.

I can remember being a child and longing to have light skin and long hair, like some of the other girls. I draped a t-shirt over my head and swung it back and forth, or twisted it into a mock ponytail. I snuck in my mom's makeup and painted on red lips so I could look more like my dolls, who all had perfect bodies, long beautiful hair, blue eyes and white faces. My mother had beautiful fair skin and long black hair. I often wondered why I didn't look more like her.

When I switched from private school to public school at the age of nine, kids picked on me and constantly harassed me because my brother and I were more academically advanced and well-mannered than most of the other students. I cringed each time my teacher made me read in front of the class. Because I used correct pronunciation and recognized all the words the other kids stumbled over, she used me as her example of what a good reader was supposed to sound like.

I read in a very fluent, descriptive manner because that was the way the nuns at Catholic school trained us to read. Even when my dad read the Bible to us, he altered his voice to fit the characters. I thought everybody read that way. It never entered my young mind that my upbringing or educational advantage would cause so much rejection and isolation from my peers.

Then, there was the fact that I studied classical piano. While the other kids were outside playing, I had to stay indoors and practice my lessons. My mother accepted nothing less than perfection, so I spent many hours separated from the other kids in the neighborhood.

When asked to accompany my elementary school choir, I pleaded with my mother to let me because I thought that would be a way to make friends. But nobody was impressed with the fact that I could play an instrument. In fact, that made it worse.

Winning the Lucy Mae Wyatt speech contest, the annual spelling bee, and getting the lead role in our school play didn't help make me popular either. I grew to hate elementary school. Although the teachers thought I was the best thing since sliced bread, the kids hated me.

Middle school was just as bad because three rival neighborhoods merged into one building. The Residence Park kids, my peers, were considered the bourgeois kids. Most of our fathers worked for Frigidaire/General Motors and were present in the home. Unlike us, a lot of kids from the other neighborhoods were from single-parent, low-income homes and they were troublemakers. Those were the days of riots, racial tension and puppy love. A lot of the time, I felt like an outsider looking in.

Once I entered high school, it was a struggle for me to get and keep a boyfriend because I wasn't allowed to have boys over. Most of the boys liked the light-skinned girls with long hair and nice bodies anyway. I certainly was not one of them. Although I was not considered fat, I did inherit the wide waistline and hips that were characteristic of the Johnson and Allman women. Skinny legs, wide hips and a wide waist didn't exactly attract teenage boys. The fact that I was inexperienced sexually didn't help one bit. I was quickly labeled as awkward, a nerd, teacher's pet and stuck up. I was cast aside by all the cool kids.

Although I didn't particularly like the bad-boy or bad-girl type in the classroom setting, I couldn't help but be intrigued by their popularity among my peers. I was so terrified of my parents and the consequences of acting up in school that I didn't dare participate in any of their foolishness. Yet, I longed to be desirable to boys and fit in with the popular girls.

It wasn't until my senior year that I had a serious relationship. It was also the first time my dad and I had conflict. I was a daddy's girl--sheltered, new to being in love, new to the hormonal changes in my body, and quick to have a hysterical meltdown about why I could not go places and do what the other kids were allowed to do. My dad probably felt like he was walking on eggshells with me, trying to balance his love for me with his parental need to protect me. I am sure he understood that he needed to allow me some freedom to grow as a young lady, but he also knew how naïve I was about teenage boys and their shenanigans. In the end, he was right. My high-school sweetheart broke my heart into a million pieces and never looked back.

For the first time in my life, I experienced such monumental heartbreak that the aftershock changed who I was and set me on a course of self-destruction, addiction and revenge that influenced nearly a decade of my life. The sad part is that on the outside, I looked like I had it all together. Nobody even suspected how deeply damaged I was, much less the fact that the cement had been poured, and the erection of my skeletal closet had begun.

7

During my college years, I filled my skeletal closet to overflowing, with dark secrets and devastating experiences that I dared not share with anyone. It was like my heart was a magnet for destructive, loveless relationships. From time to time, I rearranged my dark trophies of despair, or pulled them out to revisit the heartache. It was usually during one of these episodes that I ate myself senseless.

I became more and more reclusive and deviant in my thinking and the way in which I viewed relationships. I played men as much as they played me. I also learned some deep lessons about the opposite sex. One eye-opener was extremely pivotal for me. Men lie. Even more devastating than that was the fact that they lie to other men about their sexual conquests.

It wasn't until I became pregnant out of wedlock in my post-collegiate days that I recognized how much I depended on food to comfort and heal me. Labeled as "easy" and a "whore" by my child's father, I distanced myself from my family and tried to keep my pregnancy a secret. These were, hands down, two of the worst mistakes I ever made in my life.

It was just too painful to explain to them how miserably I had failed at yet another relationship. The fact that I thought I could hide a child was a pretty good indicator of how dysfunctional I was at the time.

For the first six months of my pregnancy, I received no prenatal care or medical guidelines regarding nutrition for me or my baby. I was too ashamed to ask for help and too stubborn to admit I knew nothing about carrying a child or preparing my body for childbirth. So, I ate whatever I craved and as often as I craved it.

By the time my baby arrived, I had packed on 70 pounds and was in the worst physical shape of my life. I was also back under my parents' roof, eating at their kitchen table. Although I didn't feel worthy of their love, support, or extravagant feasts anymore, I did appreciate their sincere attempts to make me and my surprise bundle feel welcomed in their home.

Having a child changes you, and I was no exception. I was a very good mother, but I had no idea that I was supposed to take some time for myself as well as the baby. Because I was not consciously working at staying fit or watching what I ate, I kept the baby weight on long after it should have been shed.

My mother encouraged me to eat often and sleep a lot to support my breastfeeding. Although I knew she secretly wanted the extra time to dote on her first grandchild, I played along and even welcomed the break. I was physically and emotionally exhausted. I was probably suffering from postpartum depression, something I never talked about. For months, I had no energy and no motivation to do much besides sleep. I tried not to think about how disappointed my parents must have been with the outcome of my life.

I would be lying if I said the second time I left my parents' home was completely different from the first time. Even being a new mother didn't exempt me from making bad decisions. I was influenced and controlled by my need to overindulge in everything. Food was no exception.

My life, though a closely guarded secret, was the perfect example of a good girl gone bad. It was like I had an alter ego who slipped out from time to time and totally demolished anything constructive I attempted to build. I call her "Cristal," and she reigned over my skeletal closet like a queen over her empire. She was hell-bent on payback, mass destruction, manipulation and annihilation of everything I considered sacred. She was mad at the world and out for revenge. There was little I could do to slow her down or keep her contained. No matter how much I desired to be disciplined, to live a quiet life, and practice moderation in all things, Cristal had an entirely different agenda. I was out of control, and only I knew it.

It wasn't long until I crossed paths with an all-girl heavy metal rock band, Custom Built. At the time, they were looking for a keyboard player. As fate would have it, Cristal nailed the audition. Thus began my life as a "rock star," and all the excesses that came along with it.

Rock star status demanded that I look the part, so I joined a few of my band mates in getting regular B12 shots and ingesting copious amounts of diet pills. Black beauties, coupled with starvation diets, marijuana use, and binge-drinking led me down a slippery slope of destruction. My overall health deteriorated at lightning speed. It wasn't long before I looked frail and felt awful. To onlookers, my life appeared edgy and glamorous; but, I was empty, numb and robotic. It seemed like my life was programmed for pain.

It took many years to subdue my alter ego and regain control of my life. I finally managed to have that quiet suburban lifestyle I had always dreamed of. For nearly two decades, marriage and motherhood provided the foundation for a peaceful and fulfilling existence for me. I had a wonderful, supportive husband and five beautiful children who meant the world to me. For the first time in my life, I felt like I was on the right track. My faith in God and His plan for my life were solid, well-defined and unshakeable.

Or so I thought...

8

The Temptations, one of Motown's most popular all-male singing groups of the 60s, once recorded a hit song called "Smiling Faces". As much as I sang that song growing up, I never heeded its warning. To me, it was just a really cool song with a nice beat. Maybe if I had paid closer attention to those prophetic lyrics, I could have saved myself some heartache and pain.

One of the first things that attract me to people, especially men, is their smile. In retrospect, that has probably been my biggest downfall. To me, a smile signifies warmth, a welcoming soul. It is the one thing that says to me, "I see you" or "Come closer." It is the unspoken invitation to look deeper. If the smile is accompanied by a set of beautiful pearly white teeth, then I am definitely interested.

I have had many years to analyze my failed relationships. I found that the common thread that runs through all of them is that I was betrayed over and over again by the heart behind the smile. I have embraced snakes, given my heart to weasels, slept with demons, and bound my spirit to wolves in sheep's clothing--all because I didn't look deep enough into the heart and motives of the person behind the smile.

My stories of betrayal could easily fill an entire series of books. Although these trysts and episodes of gullibility didn't occur without my participation, I was blindsided in most instances because of my unwavering trust for the other person.

I have learned, a little too late, that people will treat you the way you allow them to treat you. Unfortunately, it is usually the person you would take a bullet for that is holding the gun. Painful as it was, life taught me to distrust first and build from there. Life also taught me to keep my circle as small as possible.

I was as guarded as ever when I met my second husband. I was also in the best physical shape of my life. For several years after the breakup of the all-girl band, I practiced vegetarianism, even going so far as to grow most of my own food. My weight was ideal. Even though I had given birth to a second child, I only gained about 30 pounds and quickly shed that while breastfeeding. My little family of three spent many hours cycling, gardening, walking, running and enjoying a physically active lifestyle. I was happy, content and drama-free.

I guess it was his smile, his adoration for my children and me, and his promises of a love that would last forever that finally caused me to allow this handsome stranger into my life. Coming off the heels of an abusive first marriage, I should have known better. I totally ignored the red flag parade that marched in and out of my consciousness during our whirlwind engagement and marriage. For lack of a better word, my decision to marry again, and so soon, was downright *stupid*.

Despite our differences, and there were many, we managed to raise three beautiful children. He never treated my two children from previous relationships like they were not his own. That was probably the strongest influence on my decision to remarry. My children adored him. He was committed to making me happy. He was responsible, caring and fun.

For nearly twenty years, we enjoyed a "pseudo-Brady Bunch" lifestyle. Our blended family seemed picture perfect. Even my parents, though skeptical of how young he was, adored him. My mother even convinced me to give up my vegetarian diet and submit to my husband's desire to eat meat.

"It's not right to tell a man he can't have meat in his own home, is it?" she asked candidly.

"Mother, you know the mere smell of meat makes me nauseous at times," I explained. "Besides, my husband loves my cooking, and I haven't heard him complain."

"Well, it's no longer about you. And maybe he's not complaining to you, but he sure does act like he misses meat when he comes over here. You have to think about his needs now. And a grown man can't live off salads. It wouldn't hurt my grandkids to eat a hamburger from time to time either. I raised you on meat, and you turned out alright," she preached relentlessly.

Feeling pressured to be a submissive wife and allow my new husband to lead the family; I dutifully laid aside my desires for his and embraced his meat and potatoes logic. Before long, my physically active lifestyle and healthy meals were replaced by movie nights and pizza deliveries.

Three kids later, I was fat and unrecognizable. But my first priority was being a great wife, a good mother, and a gracious hostess to family and friends. My husband assured me that he loved me just the way I was, and vowed he would never leave me and the children. We built a strong family unit based on mutual respect, love for one another, hard work and common goals.

Our home was a loving, stable environment for our children and a sanctuary for family and friends. In many ways, our little family reminded me of my parents' home and my upbringing. We had the same number of children, both parents in the home, a dad who loved to grill, a mom doing her thing in the kitchen, and the house always full of friends and family.

The fact that my parents divorced after 30 years of marriage was something I dismissed every time the thought came back to me. "My marriage would be different" became my mantra. I guess if you say something long enough, you begin to believe it. I kept on saying that my husband only had eyes for me.

"He only has eyes for me," I chanted in my dreams, as I clicked my imaginary red-sequined pumps.

9

What is soft, wickedly sweet, melts in your mouth, and best served hot? A Krispy Kreme® donut! Even now, my mouth waters at the mention of them. I had a love affair with Krispy Kreme donuts for well over a year. They were part of my Saturday morning ritual. I was the coolest mom and wife in the world when I came home with several boxes of assorted donuts from Entenmann's Bakery Outlet and a baker's dozen of warm Krispy Kreme donuts.

I tried to only eat one or two, but I usually ended up eating four or five. Give me a piping hot cup of coffee on the side, and you would have thought I had died and gone to Heaven. I actually licked my fingers and picked up the bits of glaze off the bottom of the box. There was no sense in throwing it away. My eyes rolled back in my head as I savored all that sugary goodness. It is almost too shameful to admit, but those donuts were orgasmic.

Unfortunately, I had the same love affair with M&M's Peanut® candy, Swedish Fish®, Red Vines®, Girl Scout Cookies, Donato's® Pizza, Wendy's® home-style chicken strips, McDonald's® fries, Sam's Club® jumbo muffins and Olive Garden's® breadsticks.

Raising small children and feeding a much younger husband, whose metabolism was turbo-charged at all times, kept me in the kitchen, grocery stores and at the all-you-can-eat buffets. Although I begged my husband to take us to restaurants that only served one plate, he explained that buffets were practical for our large family and his big appetite. That was easy for him to say since he burned off his calories at his job, playing basketball, washing our cars and doing yard work.

His need to be thrifty certainly made sense to me, but my weight was spiraling out of control. Although the kids were always elated to go to the place where they could make their own ice cream sundaes, I knew this little weekend ritual was not going to turn out well for me if I kept it up.

As hard as I tried to eat small portions, I found myself sampling all fifty items on the buffet! I tried to rationalize my lack of self-control by telling myself that I was being submissive to my husband, honoring his wishes to create a pleasant weekly ritual. After all, he worked hard all week, and he thoroughly enjoyed this time with his family. He probably thought he was doing me a favor by getting me out of the kitchen for the day. It seemed downright disrespectful not to have seconds when my husband was paying for us to eat all we wanted. So I put on my happy face, and went through the buffet line again.

It was nauseating to see how much food was consumed and wasted in one place. Most of the people in there had no business being there, including me. I would sit there, stuffed and uncomfortable, while my husband and children seemed to be having the time of their lives.

As soon as we got home, we all succumbed to the dreaded food coma. Sometimes the kids fell asleep on the car ride home. I was always thankful my husband did most of the driving because I was usually too stuffed to move.

Other than household chores, shopping, running errands and chasing after the kids, I wasn't following any type of purposeful exercise program or setting aside any time for me. I became this sedentary person, with little to no motivation to work out, and certainly not enough energy to fight with my husband about adapting a healthier lifestyle for our family.

Even though I missed the exhilaration of being physically active and the energy I had when I was a much smaller size, I convinced myself that I was happy and fulfilled as long as my family had everything they needed. I constantly reminded myself that I had plenty of time to get back to my active lifestyle once the children were grown and out of the house. In light of their continuing need for my time, my desire to slim down and get fit seemed selfish and vain. It certainly didn't rank high on my list of priorities.

Looking around at my circle of lady friends and family, I was in good company. Every one of us was overweight, some more than others. We all attributed the weight gain to having children, husbands, jobs and lack of time for ourselves. All of these were legitimate reasons for packing on a few unwanted pounds, yet no one seemed to be obsessing over it. We talked often among ourselves about starting an exercise program or joining a gym, but no one was running with the ball just yet. Usually the subject switched back pretty quickly to our children and husbands.

Over time, my children became more active in sports and extra-curricular activities. My husband started working a lot of overtime, and I became a grandmother. My goal of carving out some 'me time' was pushed further underneath the pile of everything else I had to do.

One day as I was going about my household chores, my grandson, who was about four at the time, asked me, "Grandma, is that a baby in your stomach?"

It took me a minute to gather my composure, but I chuckled and said, "No, baby. Grandma is just fat."

"Oh," he said, looking a little puzzled. "It looks like a baby."

He went right on back to playing with his toys, not giving his comment a second thought. I, on the other hand, could not shake the disgusting feeling I had in the pit of my stomach. Though I wanted to burst into tears, I continued working as though the arrow of innocence had not just split my heart wide open. Stoically, I lifted my head a little higher as I fought back the tears. I was sure if I looked down, I would see blood seeping through my shirt.

10

"Every day we wake up to a world filled with people who wear masks. Like the elephant in the room, the mask is not to be acknowledged. Nor is the reason for putting it on to be disclosed. It is our duty to see that life goes on, uninterrupted and unhindered. We are soldiers. We are warriors. We are mothers. Our mission is to get the job done."

- Gwen Allman

C hildren say the darnedest things, but because their truths are packaged so nicely in innocent wrappings, we are able to assimilate them a little better than if spoken by an adult. I took my grandson's words to heart and started exercising. Before you start to shout and think this is where my story turns to triumph over defeat, let me just say that I watched a lot of exercise videos while relaxing on the couch, eating microwave kettle corn. My on-again, off-again romance with exercise was equally frustrating and short-lived.

I can't tell you how many times I purchased new gym shoes, an exercise outfit, or a fat-blaster cardio tape to no avail. Most days, I sat around the house or did my household chores dressed like I was preparing to run a marathon, not once breaking a sweat. Only now am I able to find the humor in my foolishness. It is a sad fact that half the people you meet in the stores or malls, who are dressed in athletic gear, are not athletic at all. Some are not even remotely active.

It was not until several years later when my husband told me I was fat and old that the truth finally hit me. Pow! With the force of a sledge hammer, those words knocked the wind out of me. Never ask someone to tell you the truth if you are not prepared to hear it. And certainly, don't ask for the truth in the middle of a heated argument. I never expected that to come out of the mouth of someone who had vowed before God to love me for better or worse.

My initial reaction was to scream every hurtful thing I could think of right back at him. My words sliced through that man like a warm knife through butter. All the rage I had built up from every hurtful event in recent years erupted from my mouth like hot lava spewing from a volcano. Once I started, there was no turning back. I kept on going until there was nothing else left to say.

Like so many relationships, over time, ours had morphed into something unrecognizable. I was never the same after my parents' deaths. I am sure living with me, in so much pain, was a huge burden on my husband. He worked extra hours to allow me to stay at home. I sought professional help through the grieving process, but the pain would not go away. I never found my way back to being the person he married.

I managed to function in a very quiet robotic manner after that dramatic episode between us. But the damage done to my heart was such that I couldn't recover quickly enough to meet his demands, the demands of my job, or even life's demands, for that matter. My world fell apart, one brick at a time. I no longer recognized the person I had become, inside or out. It was like one day I woke up, and I just didn't care anymore. "Dead woman walking" was written all over my soul.

Not long after that, my husband walked out the door to go to work and never returned. He left me with the children and a home that was in foreclosure. I had no choice then but to survive. My children needed a hero, and I was the only one remotely fitting that description.

11

"Strength comes when you run out of weak," I told myself, repeating it over and over again.

To be honest, I don't know how I survived my meltdown that day, but I did. I can't tell you how long I cried or laid there on the floor, but I eventually got up. The flashbacks of my tortured past could have sent me into a dark hole that I never emerged from. But I managed to pick myself up from the floor, dry my tears, take a deep cleansing breath, and shout to the face that stared back from the mirror.

"I refuse to give up and die! I refuse to do that to my children or to myself! I'm not you, Mother! I will fight for my life and my sanity! It's not over until I win!" I screamed at the image in the mirror.

I straightened my back, squared my shoulders and stood tall for the first time in years. Even though I didn't have an immediate plan of action, I knew I had to do something about my weight. I knew that being obese was at the root of my depression and low self-esteem. I knew I had to fix it, and I needed to fix it now!

I called my doctor to ask for help. Once again I found myself in that same examination room. This time, I was sure he was going to pull out the big guns--diet pills, a B12 shot, or some other magic potion that was going to magically melt every ounce of my fat away.

"I see you've picked up some weight since your last visit," he began, flipping through my chart.

"Yes, yes I have," I answered, clearing my throat. "I'm really having a hard time right now. I'm still dealing with grief and depression. To be honest, I just don't have motivation to start a diet."

"How about walking?" he asked. "I think we talked about it before. Even without dieting, just walking thirty minutes a day will help you feel a lot better."

I could feel myself turning into Medusa, the multi-headed monster of Greek mythology. As I listened to his lecture about the consequences of being obese, my family history, and how beginning a diet and a walking program could help turn things around for me, little screaming monsters filled my head and threatened to spill out of my mouth. I listened as best I could, and prayed he could not see beyond my expressionless face.

"I know you're right, Dr. McHenry. But I was hoping you could give me something to help me get started," I said. I did not dare mention diet pills, although I was hoping he would bring it up.

"Didn't I give you a copy of the American Heart Association diet the last time you were here?" he asked.

"I can't remember," I lied.

"It's a sensible eating program that will help you lose weight when combined with moderate exercise," he explained, signaling the nurse to bring me another brochure. "Just so you know, it's going to be a little more difficult to lose weight while you're taking anti-depressants, but it's not impossible. Give it a try, and I'd like to see you back in six weeks."

I reluctantly accepted the brochure, thinking to myself, "Why did I even bother to think he would understand? Where are the quacks that pass out diet pill samples and prescriptions for heavy-duty fat-burners?"

I thanked him, paid the receptionist, and headed out to my car. I paused at the trash can, but decided against it this time. Out of all the physicians in the world, why was mine one of those by-the-book types, upstanding and honest?

The battle ensued inside my car. On one hand, I knew everything my doctor said was true. On the other hand, he had said exactly the same thing the last time he saw me. I could feel my frustration bubbling up like a cauldron of hot liquid. Déjà vu was fighting to take over. To make matters worse, I was resisting the urge for a cronut and double latte with everything that was within me.

I breathed a sigh of relief as I breezed past the gas station. "I can do this," I told myself half-heartedly.

At least it was a start. I must have repeated that phrase a hundred times on the ride home. I can't understand, for the life of me, why nothing ever comes easy for me. Experience has taught me that victory is short-lived, but disappointment and defeat seem to drag on forever. Clearly, this was no different. The struggle in my head had already begun.

"Do I start my diet today, or do I wait until I eat up all the junk food in the cabinets? Should I throw away perfectly good food, or should I try to find someone to give it to? Should I walk today, or wait until I buy new walking shoes? Should I try to find an exercise buddy, or go walking alone? Do I even have any comfortable clothes to walk in? Should I walk around the neighborhood, or go to the park? Do I need a pedometer to keep track of my steps?"

The more my mind raced, the more overwhelmed I became. Rage threatened to erupt inside of me. But this time, my rage was directed at the voice inside my head that was trying to convince me I could not do this. By the time I reached home, I was having an Incredible Hulk moment, for sure.

Fueled by something supernatural, I laced up my old gym shoes, cranked the decibels on my iPod to ignorant levels, grabbed my dogs' leashes and headed back out the front door. I was on the move! It felt extremely awkward trying to coordinate the dogs with my urgent pace, but it didn't take long before they fell into rhythm beside me. I can only imagine the conversation they were having with each other.

"Mom's lost her mind, ya think?" Wisdom panted inquisitively.

"Yeah, but this is fun. I was so tired of lying around the house," Zion added, grinning from ear to ear.

"Woo hoo!" They both hurried along beside me, their little legs a blur as they raced to keep up.

I walked for over an hour that first day. I don't know if the anger was driving me or the music pumping through my headphones, but I was moving like a mad woman on a mission. I was convinced I was possessed because I couldn't remember the last time I walked across the street, let alone downtown and back. A whopping four miles!

The next day, I did the same thing. I continued walking every day for an entire month. Whenever my dogs saw me get the leashes, they leaped up and down like little Mexican jumping beans. Strangely, I felt exhilarated. I actually looked forward to my daily walks.

I decided to just hang my car keys up and act like I didn't own a car. As much as I hated to admit it, my doctor was right. In no time, I was hooked on the feeling of moving my feet. I saw things around my neighborhood in a whole new light. For the first time, I noticed how beautiful the flowers were and how breathtaking the blue hues of the sky were. I was amazed at the impressive architectural detailing on the old-world homes nearby. I can't begin to tell you the adventures me and my dogs had in that first month. It was just like college again. I had resurrected the endorphin high!

It was around the time I became acclimated to my daily walks that I heard an advertisement on TV for the upcoming American Heart Association 5K. I had no idea how long a 5K was, but I knew I wanted to do it. I figured I owed the organization that much for throwing away their diet plan when my doctor initially gave it to me. To be honest, I still wasn't following their plan to the letter, but I started eating healthier, watching my portion sizes, and drinking lots of water. I also switched to six mini-meals a day instead of three large meals.

When I found out that a 5K was a 3.1-mile run, I almost nixed the idea. I knew that I could walk at least four miles, but I had never tried running that far. Could I do it? I was extremely nervous because I couldn't think of one person in my circle that was doing this kind of stuff. Without my dogs, I wasn't sure if I could complete the distance, but I was willing to try.

I got a lukewarm response from my children when I made the big announcement that I had signed up for a 5K run. I can't say that I really blamed them. They never said it out loud, but I am sure they didn't believe I could or would really complete a 5K.

The days leading up to the event were agonizing for me. Although I continued my daily walks with my dogs, I had to fight to keep it together. I was also trying to wean myself from the anti-depressants I had taken for years, so my emotions were all over the place. The inner struggle was brutal. Fear of the unknown, low self-esteem and feelings of abandonment all weighed on me constantly.

Tears streamed down my face as cars passed me on the street. I wondered if anyone knew I was crying behind the dark sunglasses I wore. Or were they too busy wondering who the fat lady was with the two dogs? I must have looked really strange to passersby.

It was difficult moving all that weight around. My entire body hurt. My legs ached. I had lost a few pounds, but I was still grossly obese. My outfits weren't matching or pretty. I sweated profusely. Nothing about me screamed glamorous or athletic, but I kept right on walking. Sometimes, it got lonely out there, but I had to do this with or without the support of family or friends.

I wasn't just walking for vanity. I was walking for my life.

12

The day of the American Heart Association 5K couldn't have been more beautiful. The sun was shining brightly when I arrived at Wright State University's Nutter Center. The air was crisp and charged with excitement. I watched as carloads of chatty couples, giggly friends who were dressed alike, and families with T-shirts honoring their loved ones hurried toward the door to registration and the opening festivities. Nervous jitters threatened to overtake me, but I slowly made my way inside.

I picked up my registration packet and made my way through the crowds of people doing Zumba, stretching and warming up. It was wild, loud and celebratory. Everyone seemed to belong to one group or another. I felt isolated and alone, although I tried to blend in as best as I could.

Draped tables lined the floor of the arena, where vendors showcased their goods and services. Organizations and businesses proudly displayed their banners, promoting good heart health and the benefits of diet and exercise. Rows and rows of bananas, apples, granola bars, pretzels and fruit juices filled several tables. Water bottles stood at attention. Free health screenings, chair massages, cooking demos, brochures, T-shirts and gift bags beckoned the crowds of participants. Joy was evident everywhere I turned.

I heard someone calling out to me. I turned to see a smiling young lady, dressed in a white smock with a name tag.

"Would you like a chair massage?" she asked cheerfully.

"Sure, why not," I said hesitantly.

"Hi, my name is Linda. I'm from the Dayton School of Medical Massage, and I'm going to get you loosened up for the race this morning. Is this your first 5K?" she asked.

"Yes it is," I replied. "I'm a little nervous. I really don't know what to expect."

"You are going to have so much fun," she explained, guiding me to her massage chair. "I'm going to help you relax and get some blood moving to your muscles. If you'll just have a seat and place your face right here. Are you comfortable?"

"I am," I replied. "Wonderful!" was all I could say as I felt every fiber of my being relax under the gentle pressure of her touch. As the music, laughter and sounds of jubilee faded into the background, my mind briefly traveled to a place of abstract beauty, peace and well-being. In that moment, strength and determination rose up in me. When I slowly opened my eyes, I knew I was ready to tackle this new challenge head-on. It was as though my spirit was telling my body, "We can do this! Yes we can!"

I briefly heard some announcements and instructions, and I merged my way into the sea of runners that were making their way out of the arena to the starting line. It wasn't until after the announcements were made that I realized I had the option to walk the 3.1-mile course. This brought a huge sense of relief to me. I adjusted my headphones and whispered a prayer, "This is for you, Daddy. Run with me, Lord Jesus."

The gunshot pierced the morning sky, and we were off. My strategy was to run as far as I could and then walk, run some more, and then walk. It all sounded good inside my head, until I realized there were so many people that I could barely move. So I relaxed and just flowed with the crowd until I could see it thinning out a bit. When I got my chance, I picked up the pace and broke into a light jog.

"This isn't so bad," I thought to myself.

No sooner had the thought escaped my mind, I realized I was running uphill. Even though the incline was not a steep one, it was steep enough for me to know I needed a new strategy as quickly as possible. My knee immediately told the rest of my body, "I quit!" I knew I was in trouble.

Looking ahead, I saw that the incline kept going for as far as I could see. All my lofty visions of me breaking through the finish line tape ahead of all the other runners flew right out the window. My iPod continued to blast my carefully programmed playlist while my mind raced frantically to come up with Plan B. Why had I not even considered a hilly terrain?

It became increasingly clear that all my walks with the dogs had not prepared me to run a 5K, but it was too late to cry over that little bit of revelation. I was in it, and I was not going to quit. I slowed my pace down considerably, allowing some of the other runners to pass by me. I knew that my recent commitment to daily exercise had strengthened my cardiovascular system enough to endure three miles of brisk walking. So I decided to go with what I knew would work. As much as I wanted to set a new record for being the fastest runner, I was going to have to be satisfied with the fact that I finished the race, and I did my best. Armed with that mindset, I pushed myself up that hill.

13

I can't tell you how happy I was to see mile marker one! The enthusiastic volunteers stationed there quickly passed out water in brightly colored bottle holders to the sweaty crowds of participants. Now that I had reached level ground, I felt a lot more confident that the worst part was behind me. I paused long enough to get a couple swallows of water down and continued on at a brisk pace, alternating between speed walking and a light jog.

I admired the manicured lawn and campus buildings of Wright State University as I passed by them. The morning sun cast long shadows on the ground before me and bathed me with warmth as the trail wound between the stately buildings. Up ahead, an open field of beautiful green grass signaled the second mile. I could see signs posted along the trail, but I was still too far away to read them. They reminded me of the luminaries I set out every New Years' Eve to line the sidewalk leading to my front porch. I smiled. I was definitely experiencing the runner's high I had read so much about…that moment or stretch in time when euphoria sets in, and your steps sync with the music you are listening to. Though sweaty and awkwardly juggling my packet, water bottle and camera, I felt a sense of exhilaration, lightness and well-being. I was thinking how awesome this would be if I were not carrying all this stuff. I knew then there would be a next time for sure.

Just about the time I slowed down to a brisk walk again, I approached the first sign which read, "We miss you, Mom." The face of a middle-aged woman stared at me as I passed by. Up ahead, the second sign was a picture of a teenage boy, clad in a bright yellow basketball jersey, whose story filled most of the board. Though my pace would not allow me to read the entire paragraph, I did see the words, "outstanding athleticism," "massive heart attack," and "sadly missed." I was moved to tears, literally, as I continued to read sign after sign, depicting the lives of loved ones who battled heart disease and lost the fight.

I was reminded of my father's heart attack and bypass surgery. I had never seen my dad look so helpless as the night he fell through the front door, clutching his chest and begging my mom and I to help him. I had no clue what was happening to him. I had never seen a person having a heart attack before. I cried the entire night, trying to console my younger siblings while my mom rushed him to the hospital. Two days later, he flat-lined while we were visiting him in the ICU. The quick response of the trauma team saved his life for the second time. But I was scarred forever. In many of my worst nightmares, I would hear the sound of that beep-less machine and the urgency in the doctors' and nurses' voices.

For years, my dad followed a strict diet and exercise program. I can remember cooking his salt-less meals and feeling sorry for him because he could no longer eat what my mother cooked for us. Gone were the Friday night fried shrimp and oyster parties I looked forward to as a kid. Although he still manned the outdoor grill in the summer, his food was always prepared separately. I cringed every time I saw him eating a salad with just a spritz of lemon juice, or saw him pass up my mom's desserts. Yet, he never complained. Looking back, I know now that the heart attack and open heart surgery scared him pretty bad. I couldn't imagine not having a dad around back then, and it certainly wasn't any easier now that I was grown with my own children. I missed him terribly.

By now, I was balling uncontrollably and desperately trying to hide the tears behind my sunglasses. I couldn't bear to look at another sign. I hadn't realized just how much heart disease was responsible for so many untimely deaths. Motivated now by a mixture of sadness, anger and sheer determination, I quickened my pace. Before long, I could see mile marker three and the finish line ahead. The crowds of cheering spectators embraced the runners as they crossed under the balloon-filled archway. Friends and families leaped and shouted, hugged, waved banners and high-fived their teammates and sweaty loved ones as they finished the course.

Disappointment gripped me as I got closer to the finish line. I knew there wouldn't be any friends or family members waiting to celebrate me. No one really believed in me, not even my children. I had started and stopped so many diet and exercise plans that any new declaration I made was greeted with sighs and blank stares. Much like the boy who cried wolf, I had worn out the few supporters I had with my repeated failures.

I couldn't think of a single person I could openly share my struggles with or this new path I had chosen. My two biggest supporters were no longer here, and I hadn't bothered to announce to anyone, outside of my immediate family members, that I would be running a 5K. My closest friend lived miles away in another state, and I didn't even share what I was doing with her because I was so afraid of failing again.

I was quickly running out of fuel. The battle between my ears was relentless. I was tired, emotionally drained, and my whole body hurt. My legs felt like Jell-O. I was sweaty, sticky and downright uncomfortable. It would have been so easy to throw in the towel. Maybe this whole thing was a really bad idea.

Then I heard a voice so clearly that I turned my head to see if he was really there. It was my dad's voice, saying, "Come on. You can do this. I see you, and I'm so proud of you."

"Daddy..." I whispered. "I can, and I will."

Supernatural strength and the will to succeed flooded my soul like a tsunami. I didn't care what my body was telling me. I was going to finish this race. It didn't matter that no one was waiting for me at the finish line. In that moment, I knew I was not alone. I never was. This race was never about me. It was about the thousands of victims living with heart disease and those who lost their lives to it. It was about making a change, making a difference in my own life and the lives of others. It was about partnering with like-minded people to educate and inspire through my journey, financial support, lifestyle changes and a testimony of overcoming adversity.

I crossed the finish line that day to the thunderous applause of total strangers. Several random people came up to high-five me, congratulate me, and tell me what a great job I did. Breathless, yet exhilarated, I realized that although we did not share the same blood, we shared a common bond:

running for a cause. What an incredible sense of accomplishment I felt in that moment!

Adrenalin continued to course through my tired body as I made my way through the crowds of people and back to my car. The sounds of victory slowly faded into the background, and I sat there for quite a while, motionless, trying to take in the whole experience. My tired eyes scanned the crowds of people, and I saw all different shapes and sizes. Not everyone was an athlete or super model. They were people just like me, people desiring to live the best life they could and influence others along the way to adopt a healthy lifestyle. Inside each one of these people was a story waiting to be told.

I knew from that moment on I would never be the same. I knew that if I remained persistent, I would defeat obesity. If I had not taken my diet and exercise program seriously before, I was certainly about to do so now. I knew my family history of obesity, heart disease, diabetes and hypertension made me a likely candidate for a heart attack or stroke. Armed with this experience and the information I had received from the various organizations represented here today, I was convinced I could make a difference in my own life and the lives of others. I pledged right then that I would lead by example and never again entertain defeat or failure.

14

Even the lukewarm reception I was greeted with when I got home couldn't dampen the fire that was burning inside of me. My daughter reluctantly agreed to take a few pictures of me in my sweaty outfit with my runner's bib on. I taped my bib to the wall in my bedroom, where I could see it every day. You would have thought it was a crown jewel or some other sacred treasure. Although it was just a piece of paper, now crumpled and damp, it represented a significant milestone to me.

I was genuinely surprised at how sore I was for several days. I walked like the Tin Man from *The Wizard of Oz*, and wondered if a can of oil would do me well in that moment. I pampered myself with rest, elevation, pain relievers and alternating warm compresses and ice. In spite of the discomfort I felt, I was chomping at the bit to sign up for the next race. I also gained a newfound respect for athletes, especially long-distance runners.

In the past, I would have never given much thought to the football player, who is repeatedly hit and pounced upon during the course of a game, or the basketball player, running up and down the court non-stop. Now I understood why locker rooms were equipped with whirlpools, saunas and massage tables. My body had taken a beating, and every muscle I had was crying out for attention and repair.

Over the next few months, I searched daily for organizations that were sponsoring 5K runs, while continuing my daily walks and jogging with my dogs. I signed up and completed the Susan G. Komen 5K Race for the Cure in Louisville, Kentucky; The American Cancer Society 5K; The Artemis Center Against Domestic Violence 5K; The Kettering Health Network Women's Wellness Walk; The Diabetes Association 5K; and more. After a while, my bedroom wall became a monument of runner's bibs and memorabilia.

I designed T-shirts and baseball caps to wear while training. On event days, I called myself "Team Allman" and proudly displayed my dad's name with my motto, "We walk/run for life." I envisioned my entire family joining me on race day and proudly wearing the apparel I created. I even purchased a large order in hopes of inspiring some of them to participate or at least to come out for support. The one thing that impressed me most at these events was seeing a large group wearing matching apparel that honored their loved ones. Whether the loved one was a survivor or deceased, it was a meaningful way to pay homage to them and keep their memory alive. Though my children have joined me on some of my runs, I have yet to see a multitude of Team Allman participants out on the trails. It is a dream I will continue to hold on to.

Days turned into months, and months became two years since the start of my journey to weight loss and good health. In that time, I enrolled in and completed the Exercise Science

Certification at Sinclair Community College, and went on to receive the Personal Trainer Certification from The American Council on Exercise. But more importantly, I was down 90 pounds! For the first time in my life, I could look in the mirror and be proud of the reflection staring back at me.

I went from a size 22/24 to a size 12/14. I still needed to lose another thirty pounds to reach my target weight, but I was more interested in being fit and healthy than watching the number on the scale. In my heart, I knew that I was on this program for life. This was a permanent lifestyle change for me, and I was never going back to my old behaviors. More than anything else, this journey taught me to love myself enough to exercise and eat right.

15

"Who are you calling obese now, doctor?" I teased as I twirled around the examination room.

"Wow! You look amazing!" Dr. McHenry replied, genuinely surprised. "What did you do?"

"I started walking just like you suggested," I began. "I must confess that I was pretty upset with you the last time I was here. I want to apologize for that and thank you for always giving it to me straight."

"Well, you're quite welcome," he nodded. "I knew you were going through a rough patch, grieving the loss of both parents. And I also knew that getting up and getting active would trigger the right chemicals in your body to counteract those depressing moods and help you lose some weight."

"Well, you were absolutely right as always," I chuckled.

"So, what can I do for you today?" he asked, glancing at my chart.

"Absolutely nothing," I happily replied. "I just wanted to stop by and show you my new body and my new attitude. Oh, and I might not need you for a while because I'm feeling absolutely fabulous!"

We laughed together, shook hands, and wished each other the best. The nurses and receptionists all did double takes as I walked past. They showered me with compliments and words of encouragement.

"Wow! You look great!"

"You look amazing!"

"Great job!"

"Keep up the good work!"

"Look at you! I'm so jealous!"

There are no words to describe the joy I felt leaving that office. I even smiled at the trash can as I walked by it. It seemed a lifetime ago since I threw the American Heart Association diet plan away and resigned myself to be obese forever. My life had changed dramatically for the better. I was on the right path to the fulfillment of my wildest dreams. Nothing seemed impossible or out of my reach. I fought obesity, and won.

EPILOGUE

It hasn't been all rainbows and rose petals since I walked out of my doctor's office that day. I have learned that success is not a straight line from A to Z. It has many twists and turns, knockdowns and risings.

Although I have managed to keep off the majority of weight I lost, there have certainly been setbacks along the way. I learned a little something about my DNA and how our bodies are affected by genetics--sometimes, in spite of our attempts to stay healthy. But I have not let the disappointments overtake the victories. I have remained persistent to be my best self, to educate and inspire others, and to lead by example--for the benefit of my children and grandchildren.

I learned it is important to love myself enough to put my needs first. I am not effective to myself or others if my body is sick or my mind is unhealthy. It has taken many years and a lot of effort to disassemble and demolish my skeletal closet. By doing so, I have been able to forgive myself for the role I played in my own self-destruction.

Loving myself also meant getting out of my second marriage, and being okay with the fact that some of us are called to walk solo through life's journey. I have had to distance myself from family and friends that were not ready or willing to accept the new me. It was certainly two of the hardest things I have had to do, but it was necessary in order to become whole and stay true to myself.

After my support system crumbled, I had to search inward and dig deep for ways to push myself forward. I found inner strength I did not even know I had when depression and loneliness came knocking on my door for one last fling. I discovered that anger is an excellent motivator, and the trail is always a good listener. The two things I cannot live without are a good pair of sneakers and an iPod.

I still relish long walks with my dog. I stop often to observe the beautiful landscapes in my city. Azure skies and cloud formations bring peace to my soul. I get outside most days just to breathe in the fresh air, no matter the season. And I hold steadfast to the belief that there is a higher power responsible for the beauty that is nature's canvas. I rest in the palm of His hand. His unconditional love for me is the source of my strength.

Gardens, marathons, open air markets, ballets, music, art galleries, reading and writing are my addictions. Exercise relaxes me like nothing else. Endorphins continue to be my drug of choice. I am open to so many new things now. My life has become a continual journey of discovery and adventure.

I continue to be a fierce competitor in the gym, weight room and on the trails. I have completed more 5K runs than I can name, moved up to 10K, and even finished a half marathon, a whopping 13.1 miles! Team Allman can still be seen walking and running for numerous causes near and dear to my heart. It is my strong desire to run a full marathon or even an ultra-marathon one of these days.

I am hopeful sometimes beyond wisdom. Life is good, and I do not take it for granted. Even in my sixties, I thoroughly enjoy my music loud and a little radical when I am out there moving my feet. Music has a way of motivating me like nothing else. When I am overwhelmed and struggling with feelings of inadequacy, music speaks for me and to me. It has pushed me to limits of physicality that I would not have achieved had my challenge been completed in silence.

Besides prayer, exercise, accompanied by a thumping play-list, remains my main source of stress relief. No matter how unmotivated I may start, I always feel better when I am done. I am a firm believer that if you still look cute after a workout, you have not done it right. Sweat, for me, is the elixir of the gods. I cannot get enough of it.

Lastly, I am passionate about cooking my own food and eating clean. I have been blessed with extraordinary cooking skills and a keen eye for presentation. I believe food is art as well as medicine, and I have been known to go above and beyond when cooking for my family and friends. I appreciate growing my own food as well as perusing the aisles of the grocery store, where I can be spotted reading labels as though they were library books. My thirst for natural remedies, healing herbs, exotic fruits and vegetables is never-ending.

All in all, I have created a life of quiet simplicity, balance, thankfulness, and giving of myself to others for the greater good of humanity. It brings me great joy and keeps me hungry for more opportunities to inspire and share my journey.

If you have laughed, shed a few tears, or found the courage within these pages to embark on your own weight loss journey, then my job is done. I pray that you have been motivated and inspired to embrace good health and internal well-being. Armed with determination and strength, you can defeat obesity in your life and become the person you were ordained to be.

I would love to hear your stories of success. They help me stay motivated and inspired.

Keep an eye out for me on the trails. I will be the one wearing the Team Allman gear and rocking the neon ear buds.

WORKS CITED

Ogden, Cynthia L, PhD, et al. "Prevalence of Childhood and Adult Obesity in the United States." <u>JAMA</u> (2014): 806-814.

READING GROUP GUIDE

What were some of the warning signs that prompted the author to seek medical advice? Have you or someone you know experienced any of these signs?

_____

_____

_____

_____

_____

What aspects of the author's life contributed to the overeating?

_____

_____

_____

_____

_____

Is overeating a learned pattern of behavior? If so, what part did the author's parents play in the development of this pattern?

_____

_____

_____

_____

_____

What part does family history play in an obesity diagnosis?

_____

_____

_____

_____

_____

Can we be genetically-predisposed to obesity? Cite instances in the book that lead you to believe we can or cannot be genetically-predisposed to obesity.

_____

_____

_____

_____

_____

How significant is stress in an obesity diagnosis? What are some of the ways the author learned to cope with stress?

_____

_____

_____

_____

_____

Have you had painful experiences that led you to binge on food?

_____

_____

_____
_____
_____

What is BMI? Why is it a significant factor in determining obesity?

_____
_____
_____
_____
_____

What were some of the author's treatment options? Why do you suppose bariatric surgery was not offered to the author or her morbidly-obese mother?

_____
_____
_____
_____
_____

How has this book inspired you?

_____
_____
_____
_____
_____

Would you recommend this book to someone suffering from food addiction? Why?

_____

_____

_____

_____

_____

ABOUT THE AUTHOR

As a certified personal trainer with the American Council on Exercise and a fitness enthusiast, Gwen Allman has inspired numerous transformations since beginning her weight loss journey. After receiving her exercise science certification from Sinclair Community College in Dayton, Ohio, Gwen became a compassionate and outspoken advocate for exercise and nutrition education for the obese and morbidly obese client. She has worked diligently with the YMCA's *Move to Lose* program; taught on the importance of sound nutrition and exercise to participants in the American Diabetes Association's educational classes; developed individualized programs for countless clients who not only struggle with body image, but with emotional issues that are at the root of their overeating; all while enthusiastically supporting the American Heart Association and the American Cancer Society with her donations and participation in their charity events.

An ardent believer in the power of your words to transform your life, Gwen has garnered the trust and respect of clients and colleagues alike, who are inspired by her determination and zeal. "I'm not content with my own personal success if I can't duplicate that same success in the lives of the people around me."

Through her Team Allman "Marathoners on a Mission" foundation and personal websites, Gwen has worked tirelessly to inspire others by openly sharing her personal stories of triumphs and defeat. Not one to hold anything back, Gwen has allowed readers and viewers inside her struggle with obesity, food addiction, relationships, and family. Her candid transparency has drawn a captive audience to her online websites. Gwen's philosophy to lead by example has made her a hero, of sorts, to those prone to believe that conquering obesity is impossible. She is determined to see an end to obesity, and the illnesses associated with it, in her lifetime.

Gwen Allman is also an accomplished classical pianist, singer, and songwriter. She has performed and traveled extensively with some of Dayton, Ohio's well-known recording artists of the 70s and 80s.

TEAM ALLMAN
"MARATHONERS ON A MISSION"

Team Allman began as a way to honor Arthur Bura Allman. He was such a simple, caring and adoring father and grandfather. Though he lost his battle to stomach cancer long before I took my first step in his name, he made an indelible impression upon me and others with his philosophy of simple living, stewardship, family first, hard work and service to community and country. His teachings were the catalyst behind my mission to walk myself into good health.

As kids, we see our parents as super heroes. We believe they can do anything, but fail. I believed my father loved me more than anything in this world. He gave me a good foundation, sound spiritual guidance, and always provided abundantly for our family. He toiled in the fields, well into his 70s, to grow our food and make sure that we were well fed and content.

He proudly served his country in the US Army, 93rd Division of the Pacific All-Black Infantry, and labored for many years at Frigidaire, a Division of General Motors Corporation, until his retirement.

What I remember most about him are the long walks he took daily in the red dirt of the Alabama forestland that he and his siblings owned. He'd walk for miles in the hot sun, on unpaved roads, proudly telling the story of his humble beginnings to anyone who would listen. And though the sprawling homestead, thriving pastures, and lush gardens are long gone, he was able to bring them to life with his words. I was never able to finish those long walks with my dad, nor was I willing to endure his lengthy storytelling sessions. I always found an excuse to turn back around and head home, leaving my father out there, in the middle of nowhere, with his memories of days gone by. What I wouldn't give today to take one more walk with him.

So, every time I lace up my sneakers and wear the Team Allman t-shirt and hat, I do it to honor him. I can sense his presence with every step I take. All the sacrifices he made for me that I just wasn't mature enough to appreciate during his lifetime are what propel me to keep putting one foot in front of the other. The pain and weariness I sometimes feel out on the trails serve as a reminder of what he must have endured, fighting the cancer that eventually claimed his life.

I run for life. I run for healing and wholeness. I run for mental clarity. I run to stay humble. I run to empower. I run to inspire others. I run to envision a world free of sickness and disease, especially obesity and cancer. I am a marathoner on a mission. I am TEAM ALLMAN.

CONTACT GWEN

Gwen is available for one-on-one and small group personal training in the Hampton Roads, VA area. She is also available to speak to your book club, organization, corporate luncheon, health fair, church or school. Please send all inquiries to:

ARTS Fitness, LLC
P.O. Box 788
Yorktown, VA 23692

www.ingramcontent.com/pod-product-compliance
Lightning Source LLC
Chambersburg PA
CBHW052059270326
41931CB00012B/2821